GINGER

MARIAN KIM

ISBN: 1508599475

ISBN-13: 978-1508599470

CONTENTS

MARIAN KIM

1

PROPERTIES

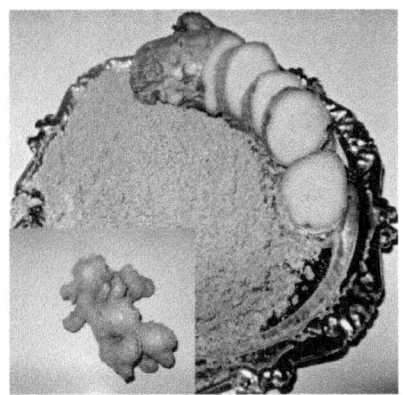

Scientific name: Zingiber officinale

Other names: Rhizome zingiberi, shoga

Properties

Anti-aging properties

Anti-cancer properties

Anti-oxidant properties which protect the cells from the free radical damage that causes premature aging and degenerative diseases

Antiseptic (antiviral, antibacterial) properties

Analgesic (pain relieving) properties

Fever reducing properties

Immune system boosting properties

* * * * *

2

USES

Medically Proven Uses

Motion sickness prevention

Ginger is used to prevent motion sickness and seasickness. Though research findings have been inconsistent, one study involving cruise ship passengers found that 500 mg ginger taken four hourly was just as effective as dimenhydrinate which is a common OTC motion sickness medication with the added advantage that it did not cause sleepiness.

Post-surgery nausea treatment

Ginger is used to treat the nausea and vomiting that develops after surgery. Studies show that taking 1 gram of ginger 1 hour before surgery can reduce the nausea and vomiting experienced by patients during the first 24 hours. Ginger oil has also been shown to prevent nausea when it is applied to the patient's wrist before surgery.

Arthritis treatment

Ginger is used to treat the pain associated with arthritis since it has anti-inflammatory properties and analgesic properties. It is also thought to decrease the pain of arthritis by increasing blood supply.

A study done in Miami revealed that ginger was effective in relieving the pain of patients with osteoarthritis. Ginger is also thought to decrease the pain associated with rheumatoid arthritis.

Therefore take half a teaspoon of ginger powder or 30 grams of fresh ginger each day. These effects of reducing the pain and swelling of arthritis are more pronounced when ginger is used together with turmeric.

Some studies also suggest that massaging the knee with oil that contains ginger and orange reduces pain and stiffness.

Menstrual pain treatment

Ginger is used to treat menstrual pain. Some studies show that ginger extract can reduce menstrual pain when taken during the monthly period.

Dyspepsia treatment

Ginger is used for upset stomachs (dyspepsia) since a study showed that taking 1.2 grams of ginger root powder 1 hour before a meal increased the rate at which food left the stomach in some people with dyspepsia.

Other Uses

Morning sickness treatment

Ginger is used to prevent the nausea and vomiting of morning sickness in some pregnant women.

Cancer related nausea treatment

Ginger is used to treat nausea related to cancer treatment.

Dizziness treatment

Ginger is used to treat dizziness.

Anorexia treatment

Ginger is used to treat anorexia or loss of appetite.

Muscle ache relief

Ginger is used to treat the pain of muscle aches.

Cellulite management

Ginger is used to manage cellulite

Migraine treatment

Ginger has pain relieving properties and it is used to treat migraines since it reduces the intensity and duration of the migraine pain when it is combined with feverfew.

Weight loss

Ginger is used for weight loss because it increase thermogenesis. This is the process by which the body produces heat and in so doing burns calories. Ginger is also said to act as an appetite suppressant by increasing satiety and thus it can help reduce caloric intake.

High blood pressure treatment

Ginger is used to treat high blood pressure since it helps regulate blood flow and this may contribute to lowering blood pressure. Ginger also prevents blood clots.

Depression treatment

Ginger has been used to treat depression for years to treat depression as an "old folks remedy".

Digestion aide

Ginger is used to aid digestion since it stimulates the flow of saliva, neutralizes acids, reduces intestinal contractions and reduces pain from flatulence/gas.

Diabetes treatment

Ginger is also used to regulate blood sugar levels.

High cholesterol treatment

Ginger has been shown to lower triglyceride and cholesterol levels in persons with high cholesterol.

Colic treatment

Ginger is used to treat colic.

Diarrhea treatment

Ginger is used to treat diarrhea.

Upper respiratory tract infection treatment

Ginger is used to treat upper respiratory tract infections. It is also used for cough and bronchitis.

Burns treatment

Juice from fresh ginger is applied to burns to treat them.

Alcohol hangover prevention

Ginger combined with brown sugar and the pith of citrus tangerine have been taken to reduce the symptoms of alcohol hangovers like nausea, vomiting and diarrhea.

Detoxification

Ginger is used for detoxification.

* * * * *

3

SAFETY PRECAUTIONS

1. Persons with bleeding disorders should not take/avoid ginger since it might increase their risk of bleeding.

2. Person with diabetes should not take/avoid ginger since it can lower blood glucose levels.

3. Persons with heart disease should not take/avoid ginger since it can worsen some heart conditions.

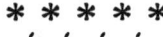

4

DRUG INTERACTIONS

1. Persons using blood thinners like coumadin (Warfarin), heparin, aspirin and other antiplatelet medications like clopidogrel (Plavix), dalteparin (Fragmin), enoxaparin (Lovenox) should avoid/not use ginger since it can slow blood clotting and cause bleeding. Other medications that can also slow blood clotting include diclofenac (Voltrare, Cataflam) and ibuprofen (Motrin, Advil).

2. Persons using diabetes medications should avoid using/not use ginger since it can lower blood sugar levels.

3. Persons using high blood pressure medications should avoid using/not use ginger since it can also lower the blood pressure and cause hypotension and an irregular heartbeat.

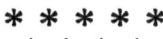

5

COOKING TIPS

Flavor: Spicy sweet

Goes well with: Poultry e.g. chicken, rice, vegetables e.g. pumpkin, asparagus and carrots, fruits e.g. bananas, pears, and citrus fruits, raisins, dates, figs, coconuts, chocolate, seafood, marinades, teas, baked desserts

Can be substituted with: Allspice, cinnamon, nutmeg

Blends well with: Allspice, anise, chives, chili pepper, cinnamon, cloves, coriander, cumin, fennel, garlic, nutmeg, onions

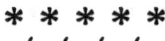

6

HERBAL RECIPES

Ginger Tea

Equipment

Tea pot or kettle

***

Ingredients

1 teaspoon of grated ginger

1 cup of boiling water

Honey to taste (optional)

***

Instructions

1. Put the ginger in a tea pot or kettle, add the boiling water and let it steep while covered for 10 -15 minutes.

2. Strain and add honey (if using) to suit your taste before drinking.

*****

Ginger Infusion

Equipment

Glass jar with tight fitting lid

***

Ingredients

1 teaspoon ginger powder or 3 teaspoons fresh, grated ginger

1 cup boiling water

***

Instructions

1. Place the ginger in the glass jar and add the boiling water.

2. Close the lid and let the mixture steep for 4 hours to 14 hours (overnight).

3. Strain the ginger and the infusion is ready for consumption.

4. Store the infusion in the refrigerator to lengthen its life.

*****

Ginger Compress

Equipment

Large bowl

Clean cloth or cotton balls

***

Ingredients

3 cups ginger infusion (see previous recipe)

***

Instructions

1. Pour the ginger infusion in the bowl.

2. Dip a clean cotton cloth in the infusion and squeeze out the excess fluid while making sure that you do not burn yourself.

3. Apply the ginger compress on the affected body part.

***

Tips

1. Ginger compresses are applied on sprains to aid their healing. Alternating hot and cold ginger compresses achieve the best results.

*****

Ginger Syrup

Equipment

Saucepan

Jar with airtight lid

***

Ingredients

1 quart (1000 ml) filtered water

1 cup peeled and sliced ginger

1 cup honey

***

Instructions

1. Place the water and ginger in a saucepan and bring to a boil.

2. Reduce the heat and let it simmer while it is partially covered until the volume is reduced to half the original volume.

3. Strain the mixture through a sieve or cheesecloth to remove the ginger.

4. Measure 1 pint (500 mls) of the liquid and add the honey.

5. Cook for a few minutes as you stir it so that it thickens.

6. Store the syrup in an airtight container in the fridge for up to 2 months.

*****

Candied Ginger

Equipment

Saucepan

Sieve

Jar with an airtight lid

***

Ingredients

1 cup of peeled and sliced ginger

3 cups of sugar

3 cups of water

***

Instructions

1. Mix the sugar and water in a saucepan and heat as you stir until the sugar dissolves.

2. Add the ginger and let the mixture boil. Let it simmer for 30-45 minutes before removing it from the heat source.

3. Strain the ginger and let it dry on wax paper for 30 minutes before storing it in an airtight container.

*****

Ginger Tincture

Equipment

Glass jar with tight fitting lid

Dark tincture bottles

Cheesecloth

***

Ingredients

14 oz (400 gm) of fresh HERB

30 oz (1 liter) of 80-100 proof vodka

***

Instructions

1. Fill 1/3 of the glass jar with the chopped ginger.

2. Add the vodka to completely fill the jar to the top.

3. Seal the jar and label it and store it in a dark place for 6 weeks ensuring that you shake them weekly.

4. After 6 weeks strain out the ginger with a cheesecloth and pour the tincture into dark tincture bottles.

5. Label the tincture bottles with the date and name of herb (ginger) used.

6. Store your herbal tinctures away from light and heat.

*****

Ginger Poultice

Equipment

Cheesecloth or old cotton sheet strips

***

Ingredients

1 tablespoon bruised, fresh ginger or powdered ginger

Boiling water

***

Instructions

1. Add enough boiling water to the ginger to wet it and make a thick paste.

2. Spoon the ginger paste onto the cheesecloth (or bed sheet strips) to make the poultice.

3. To use, apply the poultice to the affected area and cover with another piece of hot, wet cloth. Replace the hot, wet cloth when it cools with another hot one to keep the poultice hot.

*****

Ginger Infused Oil

Equipment

Double boiler

Large glass bowl

Sieve and cheesecloth

Sterilized dark jars

***

Ingredients

16 fl oz. (500 ml) vegetable oil like olive or sweet almond oil

16 oz. (500 grams) slightly bruised, fresh ginger

***

Instructions

1. Place the ginger and oil in the glass bowl ensuring that the oil covers the ginger. Simmer them in a double boiler for 1 hour at around 120 degrees Fahrenheit (49 degrees Celsius). Do not let the mixture boil. You can repeat this step several times after letting the oils cool to create more concentrated herb infused oils.

2. Strain the mixture through the sieve and cheesecloth into a clean jar as you squeeze out as much oil as you can from the cheesecloth.

3. Label your jars and store your ginger infused oils in a cool dark place or in the refrigerator and use them within 3 months.

*****

Ginger Salve

Equipment
Double boiler

Large glass bowl

Sterilized dark jars or tins

***

Ingredients
8 oz. (250 ml or 1 cup) ginger infused vegetable oil (see previous recipe)

1 oz. (30 grams) beeswax

10 drops essential oils like lavender or ginger essential oil (optional natural fragrance)

***

Instructions
1. Place the beeswax and ginger infused oil in the glass bowl and melt them in a double boiler.

2. Once melted remove from the heat source, allow to cool and add the essential oils (if using).

3. Pour the melted oils into the storage jars or tins and allow to cool completely.

4. Store the salves in a cool dark place.

*****

Ginger Butter

Equipment

Large glass bowl

Electric mixer or stick blender or wire whisk

Molds such as ice cube trays (optional)

***

Ingredients

½ cup butter

2 tablespoons of finely minced, fresh ginger

***

Instructions

1. Place the butter in a warm place so that it can soften.

2. Put butter and ginger in a large glass bowl and blend well until thoroughly mixed.

3. Refrigerate until it hardens. You can refrigerate it in molds or ice cube trays to give it a special shape.

*****

Ginger Vinegar

Equipment

Large glass bottle with a well-fitting, non-metal lid or cork

***

Ingredients

1 quart (1 liter) white vinegar

2 tablespoons of bruised, fresh ginger

***

Instructions

1. Place the ginger in the glass bottle.

2. Add the vinegar and fill the bottle to ½ inch from the top ensuring all the HERB is covered by vinegar.

3. Seal the bottle and let it stand for 6 weeks to 6 months. The longer it stands, the stronger the flavor becomes.

###

ABOUT THE AUTHOR

Marian Kim is an experienced alternative medicine practitioner.

*****

OTHER BOOKS BY THE AUTHOR

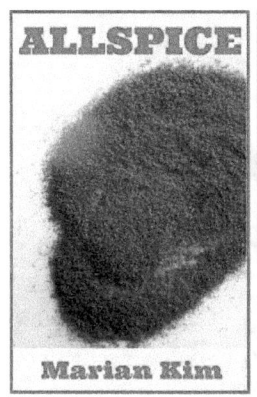

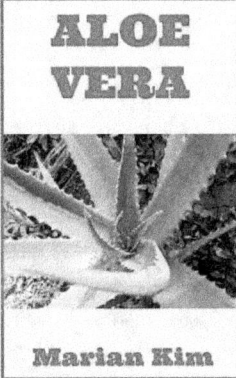

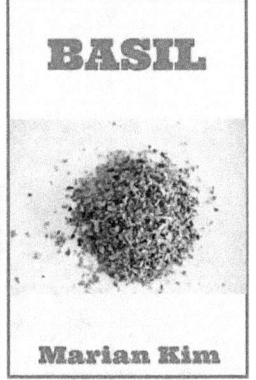

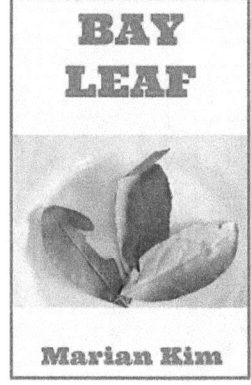

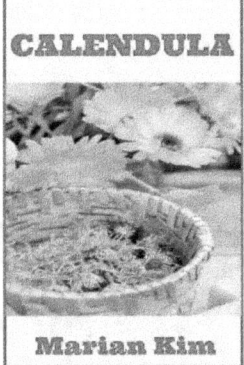

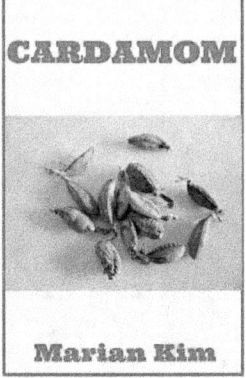

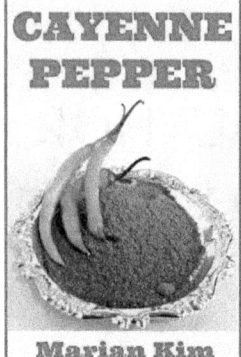

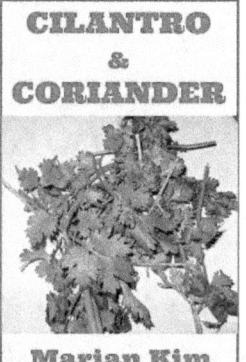

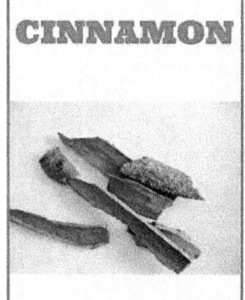

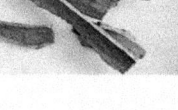

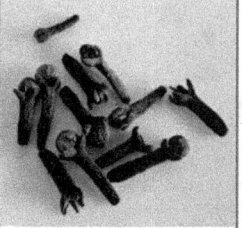

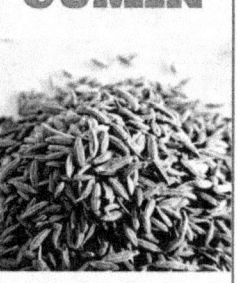

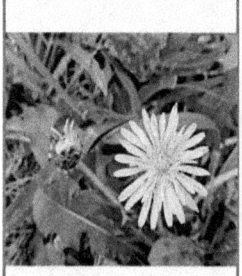

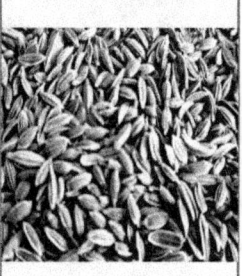

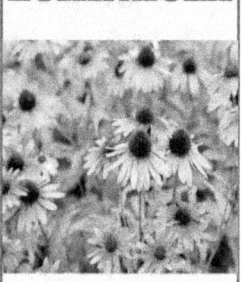

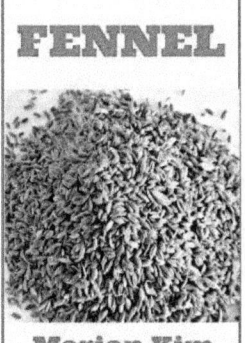

FENNEL

Marian Kim

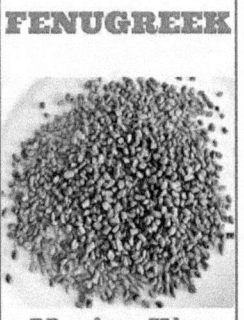

FENUGREEK

Marian Kim

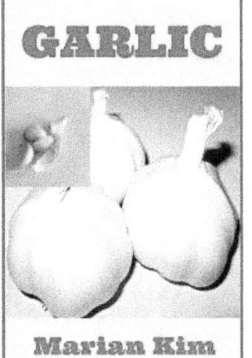

GARLIC

Marian Kim

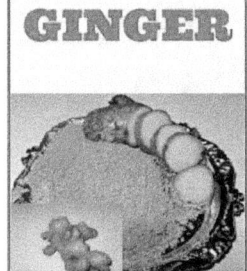

GINGER

Marian Kim

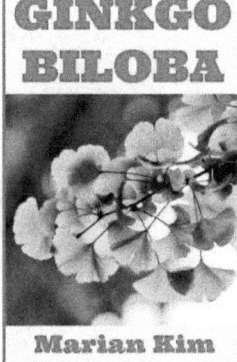

GINKGO BILOBA

Marian Kim

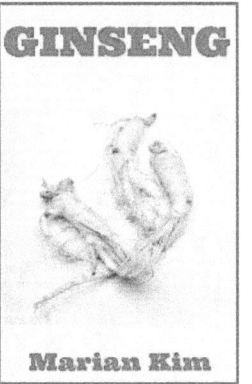

GINSENG

Marian Kim

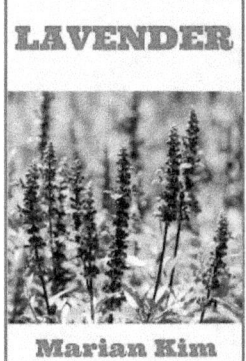

LAVENDER

Marian Kim

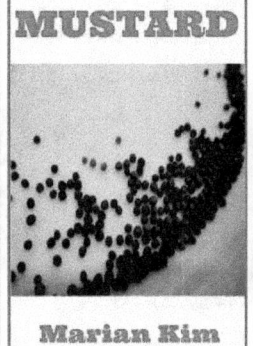

MUSTARD

Marian Kim

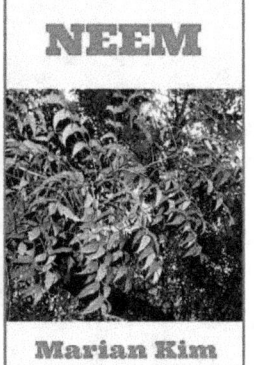

NEEM

Marian Kim

NUTMEG & MACE

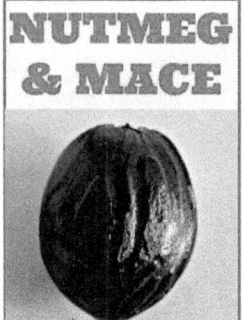

Marian Kim

OREGANO

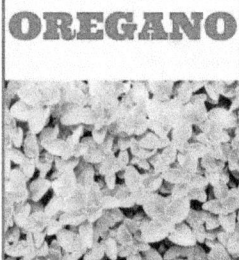

Marian Kim

PAPRIKA

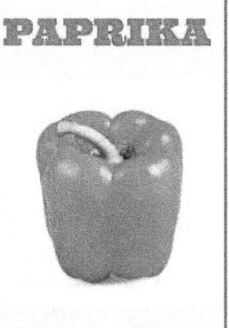

Marian Kim

PARSLEY

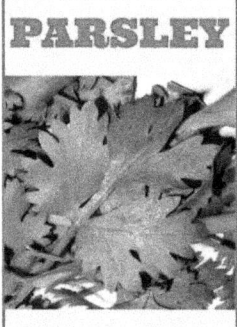

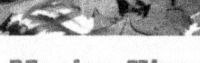

Marian Kim

BLACK & WHITE PEPPER

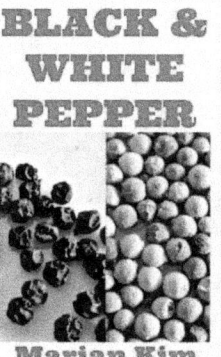

Marian Kim

PEPPERMINT

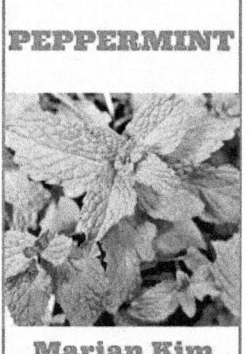

Marian Kim

ROSE HIPS

Marian Kim

ROSE PETALS

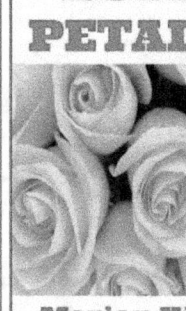

Marian Kim

ROSEMARY

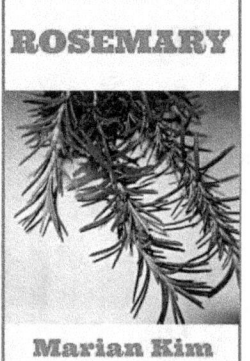

Marian Kim

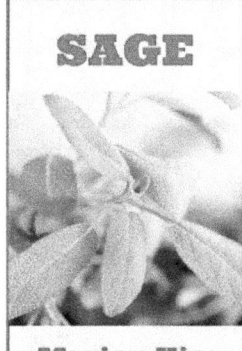

SAGE

Marian Kim

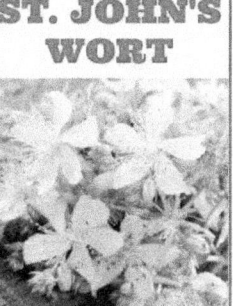

ST. JOHN'S WORT

Marian Kim

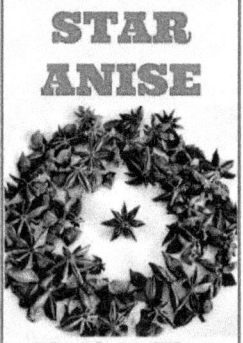

STAR ANISE

Marian Kim

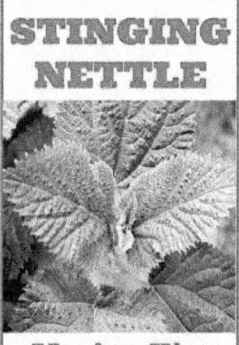

STINGING NETTLE

Marian Kim

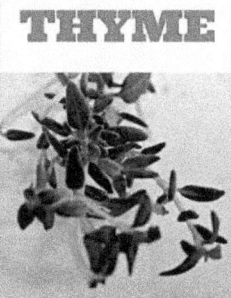

THYME

Marian Kim

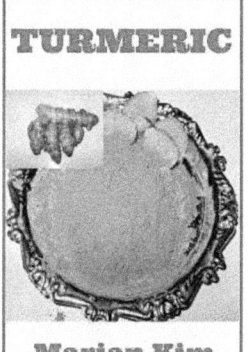

TURMERIC

Marian Kim

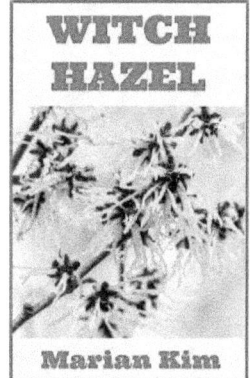

WITCH HAZEL

Marian Kim

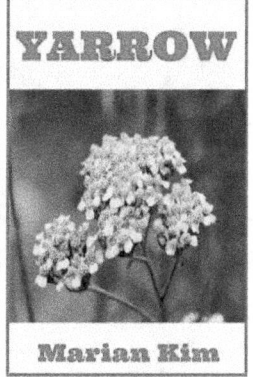

YARROW

Marian Kim

*****